YOGA FOR ANY SOUL

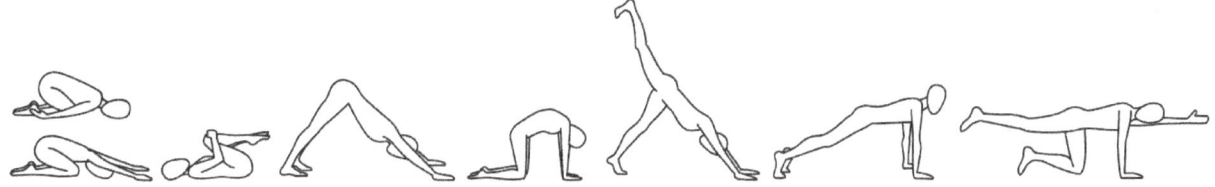

By

Maria Long

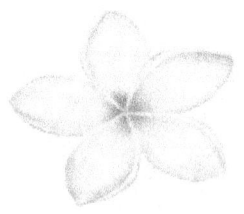

I dedicate this book

To you

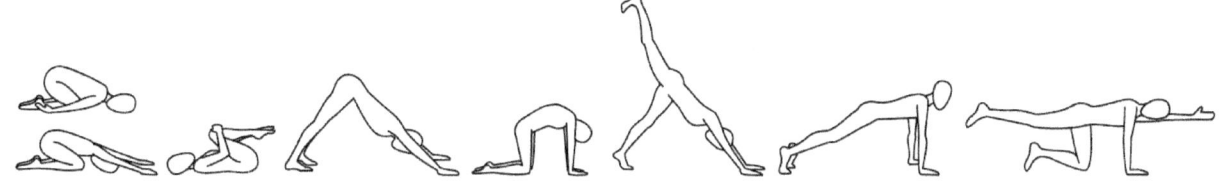

~ YOGA METHODS

~ YOGA POSES SUMMARY

~WARM UP SECTION:

    CHILD POSE

    KNEE TO CHEST POSE

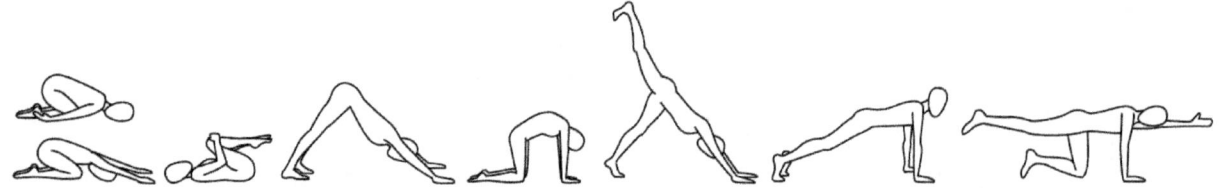

~ MAIN SECTION:

DOWNWARD DOG POSE

CAT POSE

DOWNWARD DOG SPLITS

BLANK POSE

HANDS AND KNEES BALANCE

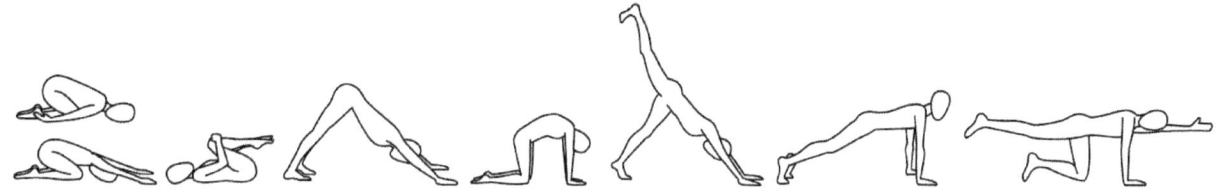

~ COOL DOWN SECTION:

    KNEE TO CHEST POSE

    CHILD POSE

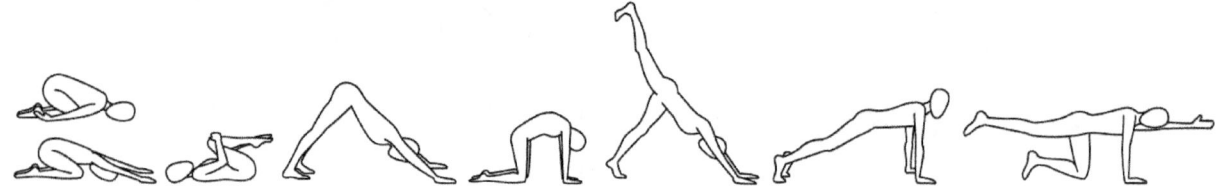

Yoga Methods

Yoga is a technique that can empower one's ability and daily skills, including flexibility, muscle toning, body strengthening, stress reducer, good blood flow, improve concentration, contributes to the digestive system and a long list of other benefits

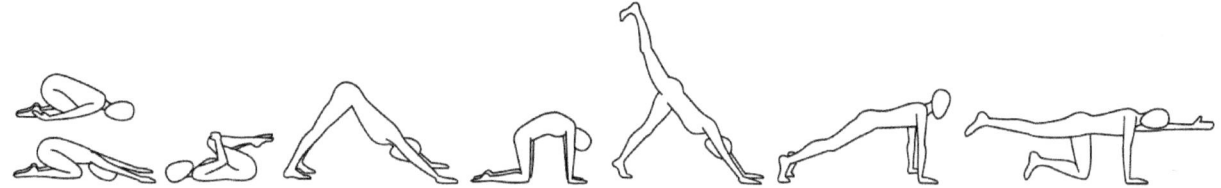

Yoga poses:

There are numerous yoga poses and positions but I find that these are the best ones to do to get a full workout and are easier for the beginner. Follow this poses in a step by step manner to get the benefits. The first part of the exercise is the warm-up section, followed by the main section and then the cool down section

Remember that yoga should be done and a slow pace and breaths should be even and steady, if you feel any discomfort you should stop doing it.

WARM UP SECTION

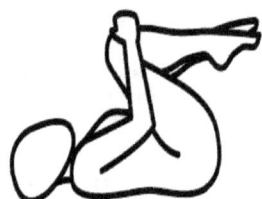

KNEE TO CHEST POSE:

Lie on a mat with arms and legs extended.

As you exhale, draw both knees to your chest hugging knees while your back is flat on the mat.

Relax shoulder blades downward towards your waist. Lower your chin slightly as if to gaze down the center of your body.

Hold for 1 minute keeping breaths smooth and even

As you exhale release and extend both legs along the floor.

Come to a resting position. Repeat 5 times.

CHILD POSE: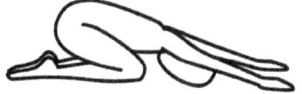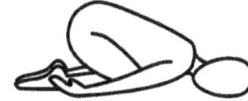

Get in a kneeling position, bring your big toes together and sit back on your heels.

Lean forward as you stretch your arms forward in front of you.

Rest your head on the mat with your arms stretched out and press your hips back towards your heels. Breathe.

Stay in this position for about 10 seconds.

Bring your arms up and get back to kneeling position.

Repeat three times.

MAIN SECTION

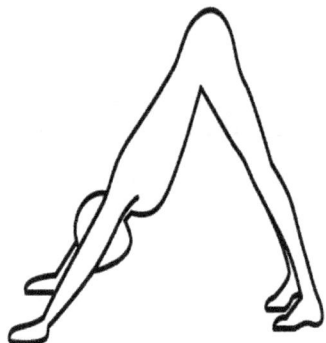

DOWNWARDDOG POSE:

Get on your hands and knees. Position your hands beneath your shoulders and your legs beneath your hips.

Curl toes under and press on mat against the balls of your feet.

Lift hips towards the ceiling until your body makes an upside down V shape.

Focus your eyes on your toes and press your heels towards the floor.

Pull your abdominal muscles in. Hold position for 5 seconds. Relax to neutral position.

Repeat 5 more times.

CAT POSE: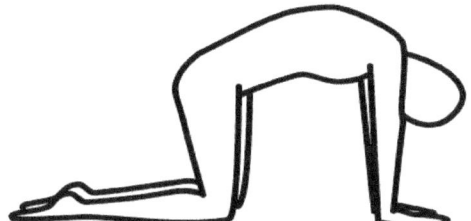

Get on hands and knees on a mat. Keep your hands directly beneath your shoulders and your knees directly beneath your hips.

Spread your fingers so the middle finger is facing forward and gaze at the floor.

Slowly inhale as you pull in your abdominal muscles. Tuck your tailbone down. Spine should be rounded upward.

Bend head inward as your looking at the floor between your knees.

Slowly exhale as you relax to neutral position on your hands and knees.

Repeat 10 times.

DOWNWARD DOG SPLITS:

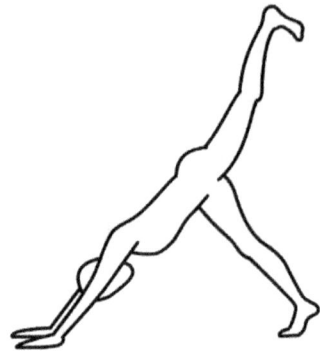

Get on your hands and knees. Position your hands beneath your shoulders and your legs beneath your hips.

Curl toes under and press on mat against the balls of your feet.

Lift hips towards the ceiling until your body makes an upside down V shape.

Focus your eyes on your toes and press your heels towards the floor.

Pull your abdominal muscles in.

Inhale. Raise your right leg in the air parallel to the floor as high as you can tolerate. Hold position for 5 seconds.

Exhale. Come back to downward dog position.

Inhale. Raise your left leg in the air parallel to the floor as high as you can tolerate. Hold position for 5 seconds.

Exhale. Come back to downward dog position.

Repeat 5 more times.

BLANK POSE:

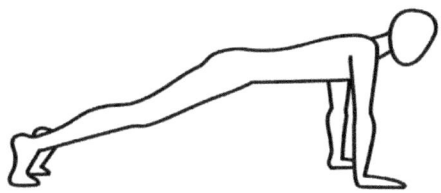

From the Cat pose neutral position extend your legs until your whole body is one straight line from the top of your head to your heels. Make sure that your bottom isn't in the air and legs are also in a straight line.

Place hands firmly in front of you and spread. Be sure that shoulders away from your ears as if in a push up position.

Neck should be in line with spine as you gaze at the floor.

Pull your abdominal muscles in.

Inhale. Hold pose for 5 seconds. Exhale as you relax and come to neutral pose.

Repeat 5 more times.

HANDS AND KNEES BALANCE:

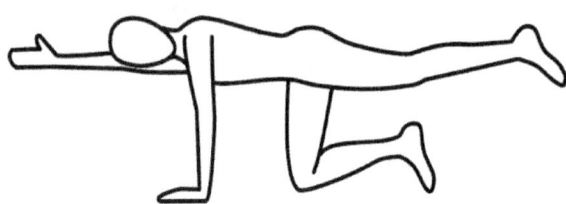

Get on your hands and knees with your spine straight.

Lift the right leg and straighten it. Stabilize the pose while leg is parallel to the floor.

When you feel stable enough raise your left arm-parallel to the floor.

Stay in hands and knees balance for 5 breaths.

Return to neutral position and work on the left side.

Lift the left leg and straighten it. Stabilize the pose while leg is parallel to the floor.

When you feel stable enough raise your right arm –parallel to the floor.

Stay in hands and knees balance for 5 breaths.

Return to neutral. Repeat for 5 minutes.

COOL DOWN SECTION

KNEE TO CHEST POSE:

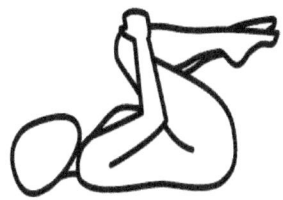

Lie on a mat with arms and legs extended.

As you exhale, draw both knees to your chest hugging knees while your back is flat on the mat.

Relax shoulder blades downward towards your waist. Lower your chin slightly as if to gaze down the center of your body.

Hold for 1 minute keeping breaths smooth and even

As you exhale release and extend both legs along the floor.

Come to a resting position. Repeat 5 times.

CHILD POSE:

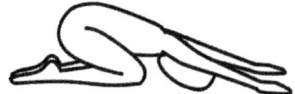 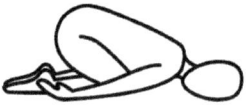

Get in a kneeling position, bring your big toes together and sit back on your heels.

Lean forward as you stretch your arms forward in front of you.

Rest your head on the mat with your arms stretched out; press your hips back towards your heels. Breathe in and out

Stay in this position for 10 seconds.

Bring your arms up and get back to kneeling position.

Repeat three times.

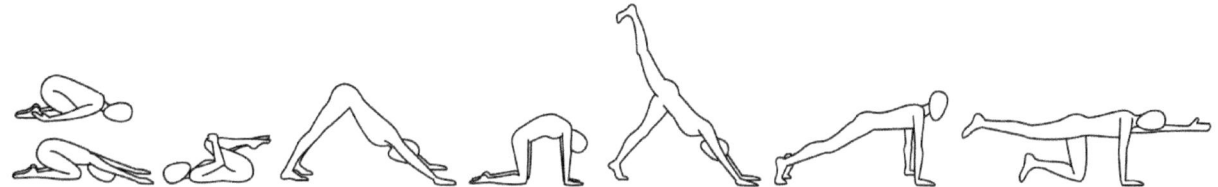

Don't let the names of these poses intimidate you. They are easy to do. The best part is that the more that you do it the easier it gets and you will be able to do them without the assistance of the book.

You know the saying: practice makes perfect. You will see results that will be very encouraging. You will feel refresh and invigorated after doing these yoga poses.

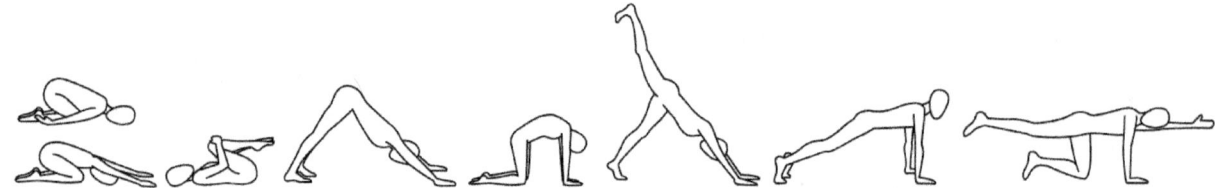

The word yoga means union, harmony and unity. Practicing yoga will help you become one with your body, mind and soul. It will help you with your breathing and consciousness.

Practicing Yoga—People have been doing yoga for thousands of years to reduce stress, gain strength, flexibility and /or to increase cardiovascular circulation. Make yoga a part of your daily routine at less once a week.

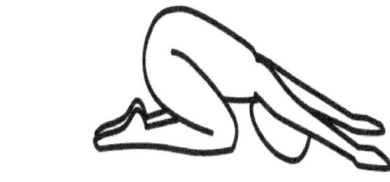

CHILD POSES

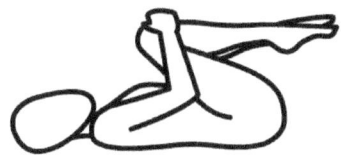

KNEE TO CHEST POSE

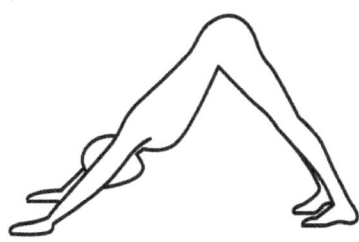

DOWNWARD DOG POSE

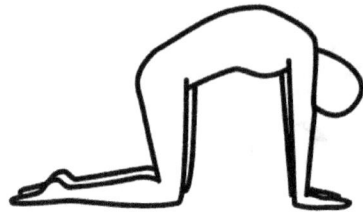

CAT POSE

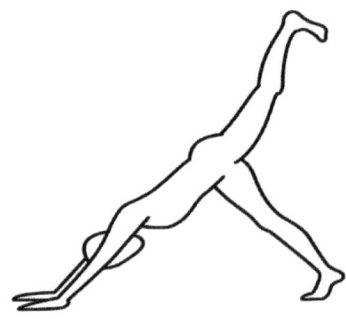

DOWNWARD DOG SPLITS

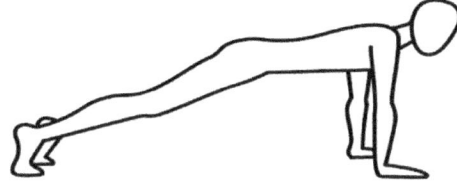

BLANK POSE

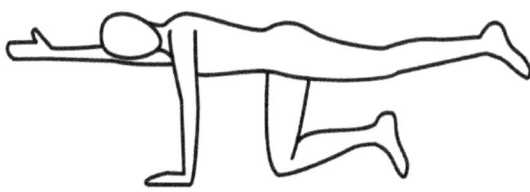

HANDS AND KNEES BALANCE

EMBRACE

PEACE

AND

JOY

About the Author

Maria Long nee Canto was born and raised in Belize City, Belize Central America. She attended St. Ignatius Catholic School. She earned her AA degree from NWFSC and attended University of West Florida in Florida. She comes from a large family and most of her relatives live in Belize City, she divides her time between Belize and Florida.

Other books include:

Affirmation for the Belizean Soul

Affirmation for the Recovering Soul

Affirmation for Any Soul

Affirmations for a Belizean Child

Affirmations for a Child

Meditation for the Belizean Soul

Meditations for Any Soul

Yoga for Any soul

Yoga for the Belizean Soul